MW00577831

The
Blissful
Breath

The Blissful Breath

10 minutes of daily breathing
exercises that will change your life

NÍALL Ó MURCHÚ

Hardie Grant

BOOKS

DEDICATION

To Josie, my companion.

Contents

'If you want to
conquer the
anxiety of life,

live in the moment,
live in the breath.

DR AMIT RAY
AUTHOR AND PHILOSOPHER

The Blissful Breath

The power of learning how to breathe with focus and intent means we can deal with stress, anxiety and fear simply, quickly and effectively.

We can find calm and control in chaos.

We can find peace and clarity despite unrelenting pressure.

We can find deep and profound experiences in the mundane.

It wasn't always like this for me, though. I suffer from asthma and I struggled and wheezed for decades.

Then my breath became my constant companion. I studied it.

Eventually, it transformed me. It made me more open and loving. It helped me to be myself.

I searched for masters who understood it.

I went to China, India and Sri Lanka looking for answers. I climbed up freezing mountains in the snow, wearing only shorts, trying to go deeper. I jumped into the sea at night. I sat and meditated in the forest. I entered states of altered consciousness, looking for it.

I searched. I experimented.

I found ways of breathing that helped me. I shared them with others. They found great benefits in them too. They shared them with more people.

My struggles with breathing ended. I was no longer wheezing.

Instead, I found the blissful breath.

The blissful breath is calming and comforting.

The blissful breath is vital and strong.

The blissful breath is restorative and redemptive.

The blissful breath is a force for good in our lives. It helps us. It heals us.

The blissful breath is when we breathe in a way that transforms us.

This is what I want to share with you.

'When the breath moves,
the mind moves.

When the breath is still,
the mind is still.'

HAṬHA YOGA PRADĪPIKĀ
A TRANSLATION AND ANALYSIS OF A 15TH-CENTURY SANSKRIT YOGIC
TEXT BY SWAMI MUKTIBODHANANDA

Finding the Blissful Breath

MY JOURNEY WITH THE BREATH

The focus on long, calming exhalations is present in many cultures. I first came across this under the watchful eye of Shifu Shi Yanzi, a world combat champion and Buddhist monk. He had been sent by the abbot of the world-famous Shaolin Temple in China to set up a temple in London. I spent many nights training outside in the rain and cold, learning how to fight. We would sprint, jump and crawl up and down a long cement ramp for hours. My muscles burned, and my lungs felt as if they were going to explode.

But then, Shifu Yanzi told us to stop and take a moment to focus on our breathing. We took deep breaths in and exhaled all the way out. Again and again. We accompanied the breathing with arm movements, reaching up and out. It helped us to grab hold of our erratic breathing and slow it down. The effect was nearly immediate: I started to feel settled and recovered; I was ready to go again, despite the cold rain and the dreaded ramp.

This was a revelation. It was the first time I had been shown that I could control how I felt by controlling my breath. I was shocked. I had been an international athlete for years, playing basketball for Ireland, but there was no attention given to our breathing and its effect on us.

Fast-forward 10 years, back in Dublin, and as I twist my body into an uncomfortable yoga position, I'm trying to stay focused on my breath. I attempt to breathe in, despite the fact my arm is wrapped around my back and I'm leaning forward over my outstretched leg. To help my mind focus on my elusive exhale, I'm encouraged to emphasise the sound the breath makes as it passes through my throat. This is known as ujjayi breath and has been used in yoga for a very long time to calm the nervous system.

Again, the effect is almost immediate. I begin to feel comfortable in the discomfort despite the sweat rolling down my back.

Jump forward another 10 years and I am in a frozen river in the mountains of Poland in the throes of winter. I'm in swimming shorts, neck-deep in bone-crunchingly cold water. I'm here as part of my training to become a Wim Hof Method instructor. I am learning how to regulate my breathing, so that I can control how I feel and think in spite of the incredibly harsh conditions.

Again, the effects of focusing on my exhale are almost immediate: the pain and shock recedes into the background; it is just me and my breath.

My journey from one discipline to the next may seem haphazard and disconnected. But there was a thread tying it all together: the breath. Specifically, if we can learn to focus on our exhale, despite the discomfort, then we can find a way to feel safe, comfortable and calm again.

YOUR JOURNEY WITH THE BREATH

How much time do you spend every day thinking about breathing?

If we stopped breathing, we'd be dead in minutes. Not in weeks and days, as with food and water, but in minutes. We could argue that breathing is the most important thing in our lives. Without it, our lives would be over very quickly.

Let's take a moment to experience this in a small way. As you read this, take a deep breath in and breathe out. Go on. Breathe in deeply and then exhale, and at the end of your exhale hold your breath. So, you have exhaled, and you are now holding your breath.

Watch what happens.

As you read this now, you'll probably feel fine as you hold your breath. But you'll start to feel a pressure build inside as you continue to hold it. You'll begin to feel a change in your body. It's beginning to adjust to the reality that you have stopped breathing. As you read this, and continue to hold your breath, you might begin to feel more pressure building in you. You might feel your throat tightening and pulsing as if you're trying to swallow.

How does it feel as the pressure builds? It might be a little unpleasant. If you can, keep holding. Our bodies have many tricks and triggers to force us to pay attention to the danger of not breathing. You're probably feeling some of them now.

When you feel a strong urge to breathe, take a deep and restorative breath in. You'll probably feel a sense of relief. You'll probably feel delighted to take that breath. Your body will certainly thank you.

It is such a relief to take that breath in.

That is just a glimpse into the incredible importance of breathing and our hunger for it. Within a minute or two of holding our breath, our entire body and mind are doing everything they can to get us started again. Our breathing is the beginning and end of our existence.

Obviously, we breathe a lot without thinking about it. About 20,000 times a day, in fact. Our autonomic nervous system breathes for us – we don't have to remember to do it. It just happens. We are built in a way that allows us to ignore our breathing completely if we want to. Most of us do.

Someone pushes us out of the way on the train and our breathing becomes erratic, reflecting our sense of shock and anger. When that unwanted email lands in our inbox, we open it fearfully and hold our breath as we read the bad news. We watch the sunrise over the sea and our breathing slows down, reflecting the openness and safety we feel. We hug someone we love, breathing in softly and dissolving into their arms as we breathe out.

Our breathing is our constant companion. It is with us through every experience: the good, the bad and the ugly. It is the one of the first things we do when we are born and one of the last when we die. It is always there with us.

Our breathing is our guide. If we were to watch it closely, it would show us how we are feeling. It is erratic when we feel worried or anxious. It is soft and smooth when we feel calm. If we watched our breathing pattern throughout any given day, we would see when we were happy and when we were frightened. It is our guide to how we are feeling and thinking.

The great news is that we can take control of our breath (when we want to).

When we feel stressed, and our breathing becomes shallow and ragged, we have a choice. In that moment, we can decide to change how we breathe. In that moment, we can decide to breathe in gently and focus on a long, smooth exhale. In that moment, we can continue to breathe like that, and we know that it will change how we feel and think.

Let's do it now as you read this.

Restorative Breathing

Breathe in gently and, without force, breathe slowly all the way out.

When you reach the end of your exhale, breathe in slowly and deeply.

Now, breathe out slowly and gently, enjoying the exhale. Allow the body to soften as you breathe. When you reach the bottom of your exhale, breathe in again. Breathe slowly.

Finally, exhale slowly and allow the muscles to soften in your jaw, your mouth and your shoulders.

This simple way of breathing will activate the vagus nerve, dropping our heart rate and moving us into the parasympathetic part of the autonomic nervous system. There, we can feel safe again. There, we can feel balanced again. There, we can feel calm again.

We have a choice in every single moment: to become aware of our breathing, to work with it to feel better, to become more open and loving.

It's time to make that choice.

This is what my book is about.

It is about changing the way you breathe. It is about changing how you feel for the better. It is about becoming the master of your own breath. This book will teach you how to do that.

It's an invaluable skill to have, especially nowadays, when many of us, myself included, are under a lot of pressure.

Simply follow the path from here to the end of the book. We'll breathe together.

You'll learn about the power and potential within each breath. You'll find time and space to practise breathing every day. You'll feel the transformative effects of taking just 10 minutes each day to practise this.

You'll come across links that will take you to guided breathing meditations.

Each way of breathing you will learn has been tested in the battleground of life. I'm not interested in ways of breathing that only work when everything is quiet, when there is no one demanding our attention or when everything is calm. Of more importance to me is learning how to breathe when we need it – no matter where we are or what circumstances we find ourselves in. We want to be able to call upon our blissful breath at any time.

We'll look at specific problems, such as stress, focus, immunity, anxiety, performance, energy, sleep, mood and recovery. We'll learn how to breathe in ways that help us to remain calm and peaceful despite the pressures we face. We'll practise for 10 minutes every day. We'll learn how to make the breathing exercises part of our day-to-day routine. We'll learn how to fit them into our already hectic schedule. We'll learn how to use our breath to transform ourselves.

If you're in desperate need of addressing one of the above problems immediately (for example, if you are feeling terribly stressed right now), then jump straight into that section. Read through it, practise the exercises and use them to change how you feel. With just 10 minutes of breathwork, you'll learn how to deal with whatever it is you are struggling with. You'll learn how to find relief and peace.

As with any skill, the more we understand it and the more we practise it, the better we become. So, once you've found relief from your struggles, I suggest you get back on the path and return to your journey of mastery.

This is where we begin now.

USING YOUR BREATH

The polyvagal theory was developed by Stephen Porges, a professor of psychiatry, and it attempts to explain how we react to everything around us – the good, the bad and the life-threatening. It is a complex theory, helping us to understand a lot of complicated things that happen inside us, but for now we only need to explore a simple version.

I live on a road of old houses that were built here in Dublin, Ireland, in the 1930s. Along the road there are often lines of parked cars and, in among the cars, my children play with their friends.

As I was driving away from our house one day, I saw a large, white SUV in my rearview mirror. At the same time, in my side mirror, I saw my youngest son coming out of our driveway, pedalling like mad in an attempt to catch up with me, so that he could say goodbye. He was oblivious to the white SUV. In a heart-stopping moment, my son flew out onto the road without looking as the SUV bore down on him. When he finally did spot it, he froze in the middle of the road. Thankfully, the SUV swerved out of the way.

But what had happened to my son? Why had he just stopped, immobile? According to polyvagal theory, this is what happens when our nervous system is faced with

a daunting emergency. His body stopped working. He felt completely overwhelmed by the situation. 'I can't do anything,' he may have thought. He felt trapped, numb and helpless. He shut down and maybe (somewhere deep inside) prepared for death.

We are going to learn how to use our breath to deal with situations like this. We'll learn how to use simple, proven and effective ways to ease our way out of this overwhelming feeling.

Let's try it now.

Box Breathing

Take a slow breath in, breathing gently up through the body. When you reach the peak of this inhalation, stop and hold your breath now for a count of two and three.

Slowly exhale (without force) and when you get to the bottom, hold your breath again for a count of two and three.

Let's do it again. Breathe in gently and slowly, breathing to the peak of your breath. Now, at the peak, stop and hold your breath for a count of two and three.

Then, slowly and softly breathe out until you reach the bottom of your exhale. Stop now and hold your breath for a count of two and three.

When we learn to follow this way of breathing, it helps us deal with overwhelming situations. It is called box breathing. We'll learn more about it later, when we discover how it can be adapted to help us in many ways.

Let's go back to my son, the SUV and the near accident on my road...

In the split second just before the SUV skidded, a lot of things happened at once. My son froze on the spot. I saw what was happening, slammed on the brakes and threw my car into reverse, shouting at my son to get out of the way. The SUV driver then saw my son, instinctively swerved, skidded and stopped.

I got out of my car and ran over to my son. I felt relief, but I also felt anger, irritation and frustration. My nervous system was ramping up, pushing me into the fight part of the fight or flight response, known as the systematic nervous system. Energy and anger were rushing through my body. My focus was becoming narrow, thinking about what could have happened – the worst-case scenario. I felt rage.

At the same time, my son was feeling something very different. He wanted to run – to get as far away from the situation as possible. He was experiencing the flight part of his nervous system's fight or flight response. He felt fear, panic and worry. He wanted to escape.

When we feel like this, whether we're in fight or flight mode, we can use our breath to change it. We can use our breath to feel safe, to feel calm, to feel connected to the people around us.

Let's try it now briefly.

Vagus Nerve Breathing

Take a moment to bring your attention to your breath as it is now. Patiently watch and listen to your breath as you inhale and exhale. Observe it for a few moments.

Now, on your next inhale, breathe in gently and breathe all the way out without force. At the bottom of the exhale, breathe in again, expanding the body as you inhale. Now breathe out slowly and steadily. Your focus is on a long and steady exhale.

Once more, breathe in, and now follow your breath as you exhale all the way out.

When we follow this way of breathing, it will bring us from a state of fight or flight down into a state where we feel calm and safe again. It is called vagus nerve breathing. We will be exploring this in more detail as we move deeper into our practice.

Eventually, things on the road settled down. I hugged my son and reassured him. We put the bike away. I parked the car, and we went inside. We talked about everything a few times over. We felt settled again, safe together. Our appetites had returned and our digestion was working again (it can be reduced when in a state of emergency). We had returned to the parasympathetic nervous system.

I felt safe. I felt open and compassionate. I was happy to be back in the house and delighted that everyone was alright. Everything was grand.

When we feel like this, our nervous system can repair and heal. We feel open and mindful. This is called the rest and digest, or rest and recover, part of the nervous system. It's governed by the parasympathetic nervous system.

Ideally, we want to be able to spend a good deal of time feeling like this. And when the stressors start to affect us, it is important that we know how to bring ourselves back down into this state of rest and recover.

We want to learn how to use our breath to feel peaceful despite these pressures. We want to use our breath to deal with stress and anxiety. We want to use our breath to improve our mood, sleep, focus and performance.

The polyvagal theory helps us understand what is going on within us as we react to the twists and turns of our daily lives. It provides a great framework to help us grasp how different levels of pressure affect us and how we can use our breathing to deal with them.

We will also explore another type of breathing called coherent breathing, which was developed by Dr Patricia L. Gerbarg and Dr Richard P. Brown, and helps us to deal better with trauma and to balance our emotions.

When we follow this way of breathing, our bodies will slip down into the parasympathetic nervous system, where we will feel safe and calm, where we can heal and repair.

Let's try it.

Coherent Breathing

Start breathing evenly in and out, measuring the length of your inhales and exhales.

Focus on the rhythm of your breath, counting the length of each inhalation and exhalation – in for six seconds and out for six seconds.

Continue in this way. You should not force or push your breath. Your lungs should find a calming pattern; your inhale should be soft and effortless, your exhale calm and peaceful.

The more you focus on this rhythm, the more balanced you will feel. Your body will let go of any tension. Your mind will open and expand.

You will feel the change.

Our breath is our companion. It is our guide.

It is our teacher.
All we have to do
now is follow it.

Stress

'If you're in a
stressful situation...

if you consciously
slow down your
breathing just for
one minute, or even
a few seconds, you
can put yourself in a
calmer state.'

LUCY NORCLIFFE-KAUFMANN
ASSOCIATE PROFESSOR OF NEUROLOGY

It was a bright evening in March 2020 and my wife, Josie, and I had just finished working around the kitchen table. We talked about our schedule for the rest of the year. Things were looking good. Tickets were selling well and most of our events would be sold out. I was delighted.

Then, it happened.

On national television, the Taoiseach (the Irish Prime Minister) announced to a stunned country that we were going into full lockdown. Nearly everything was going to shut down for weeks.

Within a few seconds, so many thoughts passed through my mind. Is this the end of our business? What will happen to us? How will we feed our four children? Will we be safe? Will we ever see our family again? Will this last forever?

Stress can be defined as what happens to us when we are thrown out of balance. The news of the unexpected and severe lockdown threw me off balance.

What happens in this situation is that the body prepares either to fight for its life or to run and hide – or it becomes immobile. In my case, my heart rate increased. There was a release of adrenalin as I prepared for danger (real or perceived). As part of that, my focus narrowed, and I started thinking about the worst-case scenario. That's anxiety, and if it was left to spiral out of control, then I would have ended up in an unholy mess.

I am sure you have experienced situations like this and reacted in a similar way.

When it happens, our breathing changes too. As we feel the pressure, our breathing becomes erratic. As the pressure builds into stress and anxiety, we might even stop breathing for a while. Or we might feel our breath coming in short, sharp bursts. Usually, though, we forget about our breathing altogether as we become focused on the worst-case scenario.

But we have a choice.

So, on that evening back in March, I decided to do just that. I made a choice. I stepped out the back door of the house, into the fresh evening air. I gently placed my attention on my breath and noticed that it was ragged and shallow. I listened to it for a moment or two and decided to change it.

I inhaled for a slow count of three and I exhaled for a slow count of six. I did it again. And again. After a few minutes, I could feel my body relax. After a few more minutes, I felt my shoulders fall and my mind start to settle. After a few more minutes, I saw that this lockdown was also an opportunity of sorts. I continued to breathe with a focus on my long exhale – vagus nerve breathing (see page 26).

After about 10 minutes of breathing like this, I felt calm and I could see that the lockdown would mean that many people would be feeling just like I was (stressed and anxious) and would need to learn how to breathe through it. I took a few more breaths and went back in to Josie and the children.

The next morning, I got a call from a marketing agency whose staff were stressed and anxious. They were worried about having to work from home, trying to balance it with home-schooling and the uncertainty that lay ahead. Could I do an online breathing class with them? It was the start of a new branch of my work: helping people all over the world to deal better with stress through their breath. I created online courses and events for them. It was an unexpected silver lining to a dark cloud.

There are many ways to breathe to deal with stress. But, from my years of teaching people how to breathe when under pressure, I have learnt a few important lessons. When we're stressed, we need something that works quickly. It also needs to be simple, so we can remember it and repeat it over and over again.

When we're under pressure, we need clear instructions.

We're going to breathe in for a count of three and breathe out for six. Nice and simple. This is a form of vagus nerve breathing.

In for three and out for six. And repeat.

Before we try it, here are a few important things to remember:

- Keep the body and breath soft and easy as you breathe.
- If you are struggling to reach a count of six on the exhale, just breathe out for as long as you can. Try breathing out for four and then, over time, you'll be able to build towards six.
- Most importantly, take it easy. Your breathing should be gentle and soft. You don't want your breathing to be another source of stress, so breathe in a comfortable way.

The Exhale

Take a moment to settle into a comfortable position, either sitting or lying down.

Place your attention gently on your breath as it is now. Don't force or change it. just quietly pay attention to it for a moment.

Now, on your next inhale, breathe in for two and three slowly, allowing the body to expand, and now breathe out slowly for a count of two, three, four, five and six.

Breathe in softly now for two and three, feeling the body expanding. Now breathe out slowly and steadily for two, three, four, five and six.

Let's do it again: breathe in slowly for a count of two and three. Now breathe out slowly and softly for two, three, four, five and six.

Slowly breathe in for two and three. Breathe out steadily and with control for two, three, four, five and six.

Last time: breathe slowly in for a count of two and three. Breathe out for the last time for two, three, four, five and six.

Pause now for a moment. Bring your attention inwards: do you maybe notice a softening in the body? A little more space between your thoughts?

If we breathe in this way five or six times, we start to feel different. Our vagus nerve starts moving us from fight or flight down into a state where we feel safe again. Our heart rate drops, our bodies start to relax and soften, and we regain a sense of calm and control. Then, at this point, our focus changes from being narrow and obsessed with the worst-case scenario to being open and expansive. This helps us to adapt to the pressure and find an answer to it.

LET'S BREATHE TOGETHER

Follow this link to practise The Exhale:
www.breathewithniall.com/blissful

Take time to practise The Exhale. Set a timer for 10 minutes and sit down and breathe with an emphasis on your exhale. Or check out the link on the previous page which will take you to a guided breathing meditation with me. Either way, you'll feel calm and peaceful afterwards. Not only that, but you will also become familiar with it. You'll get used to it. You'll remember it. Then, it becomes invaluable. Why?

During our day, pressure and stress will find us. When it does, you'll remember this exercise because you'll have practised it already. Then, you'll be able to focus on your exhale and begin to take control of how you are feeling.

It doesn't have to be a big deal: you can do it wherever you are, quietly and to yourself. Maybe you're in a meeting. Maybe you're in the supermarket. Maybe you're driving. Just bring your attention to your breath. Find your exhale. Focus on it. Elongate it and continue to breathe like this until you feel like yourself again. This is the transformative power of vagus nerve breathing.

For me, the most important part of breathing like this is using it every day to help me deal with stress and pressure. It can be an invaluable tool in our search for peace and happiness. So, we're going to practise it again now and use it to release tension from the body as well.

The Exhale exercise is great for really letting go of the stress that can build up in the body. I like to think about stress like an old coat. We go around collecting these old coats and putting them on, layer upon layer. Stress like that can suffocate us. So, use this exercise when you feel tight and stiff. Use it to wind down after a demanding activity. Use it to prepare for something difficult. When we feel loose and relaxed, we perform better, no matter what that performance is. Breathe in, exhale and soften the body: simple and effective.

Vagus nerve breathing (in its many forms) has helped millions of people around the world.

Use this type of breathing when you need it.

Use it when you feel stressed.

Use it to find peace and calm despite the pressure.

EXERCISE

The
Softening

Breathe in slowly, feeling the belly expand gently. Go on, try it; don't be shy. Breathe in slowly and now breathe all the way out.

Breathe in slowly again and breathe all the way out, following your exhale with your mind. Don't force the exhale or try to push out every last drop of your breath, just come naturally to the end and then begin to breathe again.

So, breathe in gently, allowing the belly to expand. Now, on your next exhale, allow your shoulders to soften, letting go of any tension they might be holding.

Breathe in again slowly. On your next exhale, allow your jaw to soften as you breathe all the way out.

Breathe in gently again. On your next long exhale, allow your belly to soften.

Breathe in gently, following the breath up through the body. As you breathe out fully, allow your knees to soften.

Breathe in slowly again. As you breathe out fully, exhale, allowing your feet and toes to soften.

Take a moment to rest now. Allow your breathing to return to its natural rhythm. Allow your body to rest. Bring your attention inwards and notice any changes within.

Notice the quality of your breath. Is it a little softer? A little more relaxed? Now, you're starting to use the blissful breath.

Focus

Good intentions are useless without steely focus behind them;

this we can learn.

I had never seen anyone like him. Before we started our session, he asked if he could do a bit of training. Without blinking he sprinted off down the coast, running 6½ miles (10 km) as if it was nothing. When he got back, he jumped up and hung from a pull-up bar. Then, without stopping or with what looked like much effort, he did 88 pull-ups in a row. That was just his warm-up. This was my first encounter with a real Olympic gold medallist in their prime. To protect his privacy, I shall call this superathlete Tony and we shall change his sport to athletics.

But Tony told me he had a real problem – and that I might be able to help him with it.

Before the start of a race, Tony had to get into position for at least 90 seconds. During those 90 seconds, his mind would start to run wild: going through what had to be done during the race, flying ahead up the track, finding potential problems, then imagining what would happen if those problems actually arose. Worse than that, Tony started to believe all those problems were getting bigger and bigger as the seconds ticked by. Those 90 seconds became torturous as he lost his focus and slipped into anxiety.

He wanted to change that.

Tony wanted those 90 seconds to be an opportunity to become more open, to become calmer and to be ready and prepared for the starting gun.

He wanted to look forward to those 90 seconds, not fear them.

So, we focused on using his exhalation to do that. We practised breathing in for a count of three and out for a count of six.

Let's do it together now, as I did with Tony.

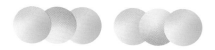

Focus on the Exhale

As you read this, breathe in slowly through the nose (if you can – otherwise, use your mouth). Now, breathe out gently for two, three, four, five and six.

Breathe in deeply and slowly for two and three. Breathe out gently for two, three, four, five and six.

As before, don't strain or force the breath if you can't reach six. Just breathe out for as long as feels comfortable for you.

We've practised this way of breathing before in the previous chapter on Stress. But to learn to keep our focus when under pressure, we must take it further.

Everything we learn in this book is designed to help you become happier and healthier despite the trials and tribulations of everyday life. These ways of breathing have been tested over and over in the heat of metaphorical battle.

Our ability to focus, despite pressure and stress, worry and fear, is a big part of that.

So, just to recap for a moment: at this stage of the journey, you have practised this vagus nerve breathing already. I hope you understand how it works (you are focusing on long exhales) and that you've experienced its calming effects. We're going to go a little deeper now. We're going to learn how to use it when the pressure comes (as it always does).

You know your body best. You know its strengths and weaknesses. Given that, you now need to make a decision. I want you to think of a physical position you can put yourself in that you find hard to maintain. We're looking for a static position that you are going to hold for a period of time that you find hard and will put pressure on you.

For example, a plank position, with your palms on the ground and your back and legs straight, with your toes holding you up. Or, maybe for you, a deep squatting position is more suitable. To do this, step your feet out so they are shoulder-width apart. Squat down, bending your knees deeply. You can put your hands straight out in front of you or wherever suits best. Stay in that position.

Or you might be reading this sitting somewhere like a bus and you can't really get up and do a plank in the aisle. So, if that is where you find yourself, discreetly slide your back up your seat a few inches, so your bum is off the seat and just hovering over it. Try to stay in this position, hovering just above your seat.

Finally, if you are reading this and you are stuck standing up somewhere, perhaps on a train, discreetly raise one foot off the ground. Try to remain balanced on one foot, with this book in your hand!

Now, stay in this position as you read on.

At the start, you'll probably feel fine. You might even be saying: 'This is easy, I'm not sure what he's on about!' But, as the seconds pass, you'll notice gravity beginning to do its job, slowly dragging you down towards the Earth's core. You'll begin to feel your muscles ache as they try to adjust and maintain the position. You may notice that you begin to lose focus and start thinking of the worst-case scenario: 'I'm going to have to let go now. I can't hold this position.'

That is the pressure we are looking for. This is just like Tony about to start his race. This is you facing the pressures in your life (in whatever form they come).

So, how to remain focused? Let's do this exercise and find out.

The Position

Maintaining the position that you have chosen, on your next inhale try to breathe in for two and three. Stay focused. Try to breathe out for six, or for as long as you can.

Perhaps you'll feel your body shaking, feeling the pressure.

Keep your attention on your breath. Focus on breathing in slowly for a count of three, and now breathe all the way out to six, if you can make it that far.

You'll notice that it's hard for your attention to stay fixed on your breath. Find your exhale and focus on it.

One last time, breathe in for two and three and now all the way out for two, three, four, five and six.

Let go. Relax. Let go of your breath, allowing your body to breathe in whatever way feels best for you.

Let your body rest. Let your breathing rest.

This is the key to being able to focus when we're strained, tired, fearful, worried or under pressure.

To be able to focus under pressure is an incredible skill to have. We can apply it to nearly everything we do. But it is a skill, and like all skills, it needs to be practised. So, if you really want to improve your focus, then get into position and practise The Position.

Not only that: I have found that one of the best ways to commit to this, and to view your progress, is to set yourself a challenge. Or, even better, I will set you a challenge! Bring to mind any activity, subject or area in which you want to improve your focus.

It might be having better focus during a specific task, or maybe during a long activity. It is up to you. It is whatever you want to improve. Rate yourself now on your level of focus at the moment:

3 = Great focus, it is always there.
2 = It comes and goes like the wind.
1 = I can't focus on anything for very long.

Write down your score. Now, I challenge you to practise The Position exercise for 10 days in a row. Every day. At the end of 10 days, observe your level of focus (and your ability to bring yourself back to focus) during your chosen activity. Give yourself a rating as before. What progress did you make? What can you improve? Keep practising.

When we practise and use this breath, we can really start to transform our lives. Imagine what it would feel like if you knew you could find a sense of calm and control in nearly any situation. Imagine what it would feel like if you knew you could feel safe again despite the stress. Imagine if you knew you could give yourself the best chance to adapt, through your breathing, to whatever life threw at you.

Then, you could be more open and loving. You could succeed. You could be yourself.

It starts with knowing that your breathing reflects what is happening to you. It starts by remembering to pay attention to your breath. It starts by finding that exhalation. It starts by breathing gently and deeply in and breathing all the way out. Then, you are beginning to master the blissful breath.

But what is the point in all of that if you're feeling run-down and sick?

Stress, focus and immunity are all connected by the golden thread of breathing. It's time to take the next step along the path: to become healthier and more resilient.

Immunity

Get into the cave now!

Your immune system
will thank you later.

I was happy. I felt blessed to have four healthy babies all under the age of four. I had a loving wife and supportive family and a job I enjoyed.

I was sitting at my desk in the offices of Concern Worldwide, a charity, with a scarf around my neck. I had on the smart casual uniform of many offices: jeans, shirt, sweater and retro trainers. But my body felt rusty. I was exhausted from all the nappy changes and late-night feeds. I was drowning under the pressure of being responsible for four little humans. I was worn out.

The scarf around my neck represented all of that. The office wasn't cold, but I was. Not because of any change in temperature, but because my mind and body were stuck in fight or flight mode. I was in a state of heightened vigilance: not from work, but from developing radar-like hearing abilities: is that one of the children crying in the night? Are they safe? Are they choking in their sleep? Many parents will have felt the same. It never turned off.

I was looking after myself as best as I could, but the cracks were beginning to show. The scarf felt like a blanket. It felt like it was keeping me warm. It felt comforting.

With the strain I was under, I would eventually get a cold. This would develop into a cough. That would develop into a chest infection, a visit to the doctor and antibiotics.

Eventually, I was sick of being sick.

The solution lay in a cave.

Kasper van der Meulen is a Dutch breathing biohacker. That means he has dedicated his life to finding ways of improving his health and happiness through a deeper understanding of breathing and science (among many other things). Kasper teaches all over the world and has guided many, many people – including myself – to make great improvements.

I once heard him talking about a cave. The story went like this...

Imagine your ancient ancestors for a moment: before mobile phones, before the Internet (imagine that), before the discovery of metal (we're going a long way back). They are settling in for the night. Your ancestors are sitting in their cave in the dark with a small fire. This is their sanctuary from the predators outside in the wilderness. This is their place to rest. They are safe here. This is their place to eat and recover.

So, that is where they are, munching on some delicacy they hunted earlier in the day.

In the cave, they are relaxed and calm. Inside their bodies, they are enjoying feelings of safety and trust. They are bonding. Their parasympathetic nervous systems are activated, their digestive systems are working on their food. For the moment, everything is peaceful. They are recuperating, healing and recovering. Their breathing is probably calm and smooth. This is their sanctuary.

Eventually, the time comes when they must leave the cave. At the mouth of the cave, they feel nervous. Outside in the wilderness there are predators, other dangers and the great unknown. As they step out of the cave and make their way into the dark forest, there are many changes taking place inside them: immediately, they become more vigilant, their bodies' nervous systems move up into fight or flight mode to deal with whatever danger is out there. Their heart rates quicken and blood rushes to their hands and feet to prepare them to fight or run.

As they move through the forest, they are on high alert.

Suddenly, there is an attack, and your ancestors plunge through the undergrowth trying to escape. They are running frantically, gasping for breath, trying to get away. Inside their bodies, much-needed energy is being diverted from their immune systems and digestive systems and is being pumped into their frantic efforts to get away. What is the point of digesting your food if you're dead? Much better to put all your effort into escaping. This is fight or flight in its absolute form: an essential part of human survival.

After a hellish pursuit, your ancestors make it back to their cave. The darkness comforts them. After a while, they start to feel safe again. Their heart rate slows, their muscles relax, their breathing becomes softer.

They light a small fire and begin to prepare their food. The smell has their mouths watering after a while. It has ignited their dormant appetites. It is time to recover and heal. The cave is their sanctuary. Here in the cave, they can recover from the attack. Here, they can heal and recuperate. Here, their immune systems can get back to protecting them and improving their health.

In some ways, not much has changed since then. When we feel safe, we begin to relax and recover. Our health improves. Likewise, when we perceive danger, we move into fight or flight mode like our ancestors did.

But there is one major change: now we often don't have a cave or a sanctuary. Even when we are in bed, before going to sleep, this sanctuary is invaded by news of political skulduggery, violence and other problems. We are distracted by notifications, comments and videos of dancing cats. They stimulate our brains, they challenge us, they push us into fight or flight mode – or they keep us up there in that heightened state.

Our sanctuary is often overridden by bleeping, pinging and flashing screens. Each flick, swipe and like triggers a reaction in us that we may not even be aware of. The constant stimulation, when added to the other pressures we face every day, means that we are outside the cave for longer and longer periods of time. We are becoming overwhelmed by stress.

I think the American Psychology Association put it as succinctly as possible with the title of a research article on immunity entitled 'Stress Weakens the Immune System' (23 February 2006).

Pretty clear, right?

Our immune systems are dampened down as levels of stress, worry and fear increase. Of course, we can deal with this in short bursts. But our health suffers if we can't get back into the cave at some point. Most of us spend too much time outside the cave.

Do you recognise this scenario?

There is good news, though: one of the best ways to rest and recover is to focus on slow, calm breathing. This reduces the stress and fear and enables us to move from outside the cave (fight or flight/sympathetic nervous system) to inside the cave (rest and digest/parasympathetic nervous system).

Let's do it now...

Prepare yourself by taking a moment to settle, sitting or lying down somewhere safe and comfortable.

Our emphasis now will be on gentle full inhales, breathing up through the body and feeling it expand. Then, when you reach the peak of your inhale, you simply let go. You release your breath, allowing the body to exhale without force. When you breathe out, you can sigh if you're comfortable with that. Or, if you prefer to breathe quietly, just let go of the breath.

When we let go of the exhale, we are also letting go of tension in the body. Each exhale is our chance to release tension, strain and worry. As we let go, as we release, we move down into the parasympathetic nervous system, we slip into the cave and there we can repair, heal and improve our immunity.

The De-stressor

As you read this, soften your shoulders, letting go of any tension you might be holding there. Begin to gently pay attention to your breath. Watch and listen to your breath as it is now. No forcing or changing it, just watching it.

Follow the breath as you inhale and exhale for a few moments.

On your next inhale, breathe softly and fully up through your body. Feel the breath expanding and filling the belly as you breathe in. When you reach the peak of your breath, just let go. Release your breath. Release any tension you might be holding in your shoulders. Just surrender and enjoy the feeling of the release.

When you feel the urge to breathe again, take a slow, deep breath in, following it to its peak. Then, just release the breath, let it all go. Surrender to the release. Surrender to the feeling. Allow your body to sag. There is nothing to hold here. Just release.

Now, breathe in slowly again, feeling the breath moving up through the body. Enjoy the feeling of expansion. Follow the breath to its peak. Then, just let it go. Release the breath. Release your body. Allow yourself to surrender and sigh.

One final time...

Breathe in, feeling your body expand, then follow the breath as it moves up through you. At its peak, just release the breath. Just release any tension you might be holding on to. Just surrender. Soften your muscles.

Sometimes, this exercise can be quite emotional. We don't often give ourselves a chance to let go, to surrender and to release. So, when we start doing it, we can feel emotional as we move a state of imbalance into balance.

Pause now for a moment and allow your breathing to find its way back to its normal rhythm. Take a moment to rest. Bring your attention inwards, noticing any changes in the body.

This exercise can really help us unwind, release tension and untangle the knots we sometimes tie ourselves up in! If we are feeling on the edge or in survival mode, our immune systems are often underperforming. High levels of stress can leave us feeling run-down, tired and sick. So, if you are feeling like that, take time every morning and evening to do this quick and simple De-stressor exercise.

Our ancestors had their caves, their sanctuaries. Their caves gave them a chance to rest and recover. They gave their immune systems a chance to recuperate. Our modern-day caves might not be as dark and restful, but we now know that we can use our breathing to find that place of recuperation and recovery when we need it.

Anxiety

'I used [this way of
breathing] every day
in SEAL training... it
helped me graduate as
the honour man, [the]
number one graduate.

Now I use it for every
challenging situation, and
practise it daily.'

MARK DIVINE
RETIRED US NAVY SEAL COMMANDER

This was my biggest opportunity yet. This would get my work out to a huge audience. This was a primetime TV show on Ireland's national broadcaster, RTÉ. It wasn't my first time on TV, but it was the most important one. I wanted it to go really well. It had to.

So there I was, standing in Platinum Gyms in Malahide, County Dublin, looking into the dark lifeless lens of a TV camera. It was like a black, unblinking eye, staring back at me. Behind it was a director, a couple of producers, another camera person, a sound person and the two stars of the show. Everyone was looking at me. The director said, 'Níall, we're going live in two minutes,' and then just waited with everyone else, looking at me.

I could feel my heart beginning to pound in my chest. I could feel my body moving into fight or flight. I could hear the thoughts beginning to swirl around in my head: 'What am I meant to say again? What am I meant to do?'

I could feel the anxiety building – would it overwhelm me in front of everyone?

But I had a choice.

Without anyone really noticing, I inhaled softly for a count of three and I stopped, holding my breath for three.

I exhaled slowly for three and held my breath again for three.

I repeated this cycle of breathing and holding for the next minute or so.

It was like I had switched on a break: my mental chatter slowed down, my body relaxed, and I could focus again. As this change took place, I remembered what my friend Stephen Flynn (the co-founder of The Happy Pear) had told me: 'Just ignore the cameras, pretend they are not there and be yourself.'

'And... action!' shouted the director, and off we went. I felt calm and blissful.

The combination of breathing with short breath-holds isn't a new phenomenon. It is present, for example, in a branch of breathing called pranayama, which is used in yoga. But in modern times, it has been rebranded and repackaged by the most unlikely of wellness experts: the US Navy SEALs (short for Sea, Air and Land Teams).

The SEALs are an elite unit within the navy that ends up in some of the most dangerous situations on Earth. They needed to find a way to deal with the turmoil that goes on inside us before we face the most life-threatening situations. For example, jumping out of planes at night over enemy territory, or running into a building packed full of armed combatants. Or, in my case, staring down the lens of a big TV camera. For most people, doing something as dangerous as jumping out of a plane at night would be overwhelming. It would be like a deer blinking in the headlights of a car – or my youngest son standing immobile in the middle of the road with the white SUV thundering towards him (see page 22).

We may not find ourselves in highly dramatic situations like this all the time. But many other everyday things (such as constant distraction, a never-ending to-do list, commuting long distances) can overwhelm us. It can be an accumulation of many small things that piles the pressure on us. We all have different struggles. What is important here is that we can all use this simple and effective way of breathing to put the brakes on the overwhelming and anxious feelings and help us find control and calm amidst the chaos.

According to the website Medical News Today: '... current studies are convincing in their evidence for box breathing as a powerful tool in managing stress, regaining focus, and encouraging positive emotions and state of mind'.

Let's try it now.

The Calming Box

Take a deep breath in and sigh as you exhale slowly. Pause for a moment, and now let's do it again. Breathe in luxuriously, enjoying your deep inhale, and now breathe out, sighing as you let go of the breath.

Take a moment to bring your attention to your mouth and jaw. Now, allow them to soften.

Take a moment to bring your attention to your shoulders. And as you read this, allow them to soften.

Take a moment to just listen to your breath as it is. No need to force or change it – just observe it.

On your next inhale, breathe in slowly for a count of two and three. Now, breathe out slowly for a count of two and three.

Slowly in again for a count of two and three. Slowly out for a count of two and three. Breathe slowly and fully in for two and three. Now, hold your breath for a count of two and three.

Slowly breathe out for a count of two and three. Now, hold your breath again for two and three.

Breathe slowly and fully in for two and three. Hold your breath now for two and three.

Exhale slowly for a count of two and three. At the bottom of your exhale, hold your breath for two and three.

Last time: let's breathe in deeply for two and three. Now, hold your breath for two and three.

Breathe out slowly now for a count of two and three. Finally, hold your breath for two and three.

Take a nice, deep breath in and exhale now with a sigh. Rest for a moment. Allow your breath to return to its natural rhythm. Allow the body to rest.

LET'S BREATHE TOGETHER

Follow this link to practise The Calming Box:
www.breathewithniall.com/blissful

You can return to The Calming Box exercise whenever you are feeling overwhelmed or anxious. Repeat it as many times as necessary to feel calm and safe again.

But, as well as that, think of it as a way of preventing anxiety from taking hold of you. If you practise this excercise for 10 minutes once a day, then you will become calm, and you'll be ready for the pressure when it comes.

Eventually, this count of three (inhaling for three, holding for three, exhaling for three and holding for three) will become comfortable for you. When it does, increase your count to four. Then, eventually to five and beyond. It is not a competition, though: keep the body and your breathing relaxed and easy as you practise this.

Chamomile

It used to fascinate me when I learnt that Zen Buddhist monks would use green tea as an aid to their meditation. The tea would help to keep them alert and focused during their long hours sitting cross-legged. I spent a decade training to be a herbalist. I wanted to know how we can use the plants that grow around us to improve our lives. In my work over the years, I could see a pattern in many of the people who came to me for help. They were anxious and worried, and it was getting worse, affecting the quality of their lives and relationships.

The monks were always in the back of my mind. How could I use plants to help these people in a similar way? That question then became: how can I use plants to help these people breathe in a better way? Eventually, I found the answer, and it is yellow and white and beautiful.

Feelings of anxiety and dread can be made worse by what we drink. Alcohol, for example. The opposite is also true. Feelings of anxiety and dread can be lessened by what we drink. Especially when we combine it with 10 minutes of Box Breathing (see page 24) every day. So, what to drink? Strong, cold chamomile tea.

According to the National Center for Biotechnology Information in the US: 'Chamomile can help in improving cardiovascular conditions, stimulate [the] immune system and provide some protection against cancer.' But here, we are using it for its calming and soothing properties. I have seen it used to great effect to relieve anxiety when combined with the breathing exercises in this chapter. Here is how to prepare some chamomile tea:

1. Place two teaspoons of dried chamomile flowers in a mug. You can also use two teabags of chamomile flowers.

2. Fill the mug with boiling water, then cover with a saucer or something similar. This helps to keep the essential oils from escaping with the steam.

3. Leave the tea to cool. Once it has cooled down, drink throughout the day.

The tea tastes extremely bitter, but when combined with these breathing exercises, it is soothing and can help unwind an agitated mind.

A black lifeless TV camera staring at us can cause worry and anxiety. A midnight parachute jump can cause fear and hesitation. I'm sure you can think of a situation in your life that feels as if it could overwhelm you. We've all been there. And we will again.

Anxiety is a natural reaction to pressure.

When we're anxious, we start thinking about the worst-case scenario. We begin to prepare mentally for it. We are built to deal with this in short bursts. Problems arise when that anxiety deepens and deepens, spiralling into a seemingly endless pattern of worst-case scenarios. It can feel like we're drowning, as if we're about to become overwhelmed.

That is when we need a brake – something to stop the slide downwards.

Breathe. Hold. Breathe. Hold.

It breaks the pattern of worst-case scenarios. It calms us down. It gets us ready.

Ready for what?

Your performance.

Performance

'When you improve
a little each day,

eventually big
things occur."

JOHN WOODEN
LEGENDARY AMERICAN BASKETBALL COACH

You step onstage and the bright lights blind you for a second. But then you step forward to the front of the stage. You feel comfortable and happy. You look out at the big crowd of people watching you, and pause to savour the moment. That atmosphere feels electric. This is it. You take a breath in and begin to talk freely, fluently with insight and humour. Everything is flowing.

Wow, wouldn't that be great? To have the poise and confidence to speak in public like that. This is a performance. Many people can do it. Many people are terrified by it.

You burst into the kitchen before you drop the heavy shopping bags you've carried from the car. You're soaking. It is raining so hard that you got wet on the short walk up the driveway. The kitchen is still a mess from this morning. You'd forgotten about that. The children will be home at any moment now, and will be 'starving', as they always tell you. You've got work to do. You've got food to make. You've got to clean the kitchen. You can feel the pressure building in your head. You've got to get them to training by 6 p.m. This is a performance.

You've a sales deadline that you have to hit. You need that bonus. Your personal finances are in chaos. That bonus will save the day. But you're behind. Your leads have dried up. The end of the sales period is just around the corner. Your team is underperforming. You can feel the pressure building. You've got to hit this deadline. This is a performance.

When people hear the word 'performance', they often think of elite athletes or someone other than themselves. But really, our whole day is a performance. We're trying to do stuff. Often successfully. Often not.

Often with ease. Often under pressure. But we are still performing.

When we feel open and calm, our focus is expansive. We can see a situation in its entirety, and we find it easy to adapt. We feel safe. Our bodies feel loose. We can handle the pressure as it comes. We adapt to it and find ways around it. We can perform well.

When we feel tense, our focus begins to narrow. The problem, the obstacle, the issue becomes our focus. We can feel unsafe and exposed. Our bodies become tight and tense. We gather pressure around us like an old coat. It is hard to take off again. It can drain our energy. It becomes harder to perform.

A friend once told me about his experiences at work. It was a high-pressure, unpleasant environment to work in. Things were getting too much for him. So, he excused himself for a minute and went to the toilet. Sitting in the toilet cubicle, he began to breathe calmly and slowly: breathing in, holding, breathing out and holding. He wasn't forcing it, just allowing his breath to come naturally without pushing. After a few minutes, he began to feel different, better. After a few more minutes, he felt calm. He was ready to go back to work. He was ready for his performance.

I felt this way many times as an international athlete. Sometimes the pressure was high, and I just flowed with it.

Everything worked perfectly well. Other times, the pressure dragged on me. It depends on loads of things, but one important part of it is our state of mind, our state of body and the state of our breath.

The greatest advantage a competitor can have is knowing that they can (at any moment) improve their state of mind and state of body by changing how they are breathing. It is that simple. But, as a wise person once said, 'It may be simple, but it is not easy.'

It is not easy to remember that in the middle of any performance, we have a choice:

We can improve our experience by improving how we breathe.

We can decide to change how we breathe and, by doing so, change how we feel and perform.

Often, we want to break the pattern of our thoughts: they might be stuck in a worrying cycle that is getting worse and worse. We want to be able to stop that, to break that cycle and replace it with a mind that is soothed and calm. We want to do that quickly.

So, let's do it.

We're going to build on the previous breathing exercise – The Calming Box (see page 72) – and go deeper.

Now I would like you to take a second to think about your most difficult performance of the day. What is the thing that makes you most anxious or worried? What is the thing you struggle with? For me, it is putting my children to bed. I know, it doesn't sound like much of a struggle, but it can be. My four children are my gurus. They teach me infinite lessons in patience, compassion, humour and love. But the lessons aren't always easy to learn.

This is what can happen: after an early start and a long and exciting day of work, the final battle is getting everyone to bed on time with their teeth brushed. Often, I might have an event later in the evening, so there is also a bit of a deadline looming. What follows can be stressful and it often really pushes me to the edge (and beyond) of my patience.

That is my example. Now I'd like you to think of the performance you want to improve.

I want you to think of the thing that feels as if it might overwhelm you. As you read this, bring to mind the details of the situation: where are you? Who is there? What time is it?

How do you feel physically? Where in your body do you feel the tension and pressure? In your jaw? Your shoulders? Your gut?

What thoughts go through your mind when the performance begins? Allow them in. Feel them.

As this struggle is in our minds, we are now going to change how we breathe and how we experience this struggle. We are going to change how we feel through our breathing. We are going to change our experience of the performance.

The Powerful Performance

As you read this, bring your attention to your breath. Place your attention on it gently. Listen to it for a moment.

With your next inhale, breathe in deeply for a count of two and three and then hold. Hold for a count of two and three.

Breathe out slowly for a count of two and three. Hold now for a count of two and three.

Breathe in deeply for a count of two and three. Hold now for two and three.

Breathe out slowly and steadily for two and three. Hold now, without force, for a count of two and three.

Allow your mind to follow the breath...

Breathe in slowly and steadily for two and three. Hold now for a count of two and three.

Breathe out slowly for two and three. Now hold your breath for a count of two and three.

Pause now for a moment.

Allow your breathing to find its way back to normal.

Bring your attention inwards for a few moments. Notice the softness of your body. Notice the gentleness of your breath. Notice the openness of your thoughts.

Bring to mind your performance now. Try to remember what it was. But now I want you to try to memorise how you feel in this moment after doing the breathing. Memorise the softness of your body. Memorise the gentleness of your breath. Memorise the openness of your thoughts, despite the struggle of the performance.

Now, let's breathe together again... twice more.

Breathe in deeply and slowly, feeling your body expanding with light and energy for two and three. Hold your breath now, feeling the energy of the breath inside you, for a count of two and three.

Release the breath, exhaling slowly and steadily and letting go of tension in the body as you exhale for a count of two and three.

Pause and hold your breath now, and release any tension you have in the shoulders, holding for a count of two and three.

Last time...

Breathe in deeply, feeling your body expanding with energy and light, and continue breathing for two and three.

Now hold your breath and feel the power of your breath inside as you hold for two and three.

Breathe out slowly, releasing any tension you might be feeling and exhaling for two and three. Finally, hold your breath now for the final count of two and three.

And let go.

You have begun to master the ability to change how you feel at will. You have done it while contemplating the performance you want to improve. This is a practice. You have done it now. When, in your daily life, this struggle begins to happen, remember this practice. You have already done it.

You have rehearsed this mentally. Your body has memorised it.

Think of the times of the day when you might struggle. These are performances that you want to improve. I'm sure you can think of a few! I definitely can.

Go back now and practise this Powerful Performance exercise with these moments in mind. When you do the exercise, really try to feel the sense of calm and control in your body. Feel your muscles soften. Notice the power and control in your breath. You are in control of your breath.

You are in control of how you are reacting. You are in control of your powerful performance. You can conquer the struggle. You can change how you feel at will. You can improve your performance at will. Memorise these feelings. Let them seep into you.

You're ready for your performance.

We are performing all the time. Sometimes in front of big crowds. Sometimes in front of a laptop screen. Sometimes when we are all alone.

The key to performing well is being in a state of mind and body that allows us to do what we need to do. We can now use our breathing to do that.

We can use our breathing to improve our focus under pressure. We can use it to deal with stress and anxiety. We can use it to strengthen our immunity. Add all of that together and your blissful breath can greatly improve your performance.

But what if we're too tired to even get started? We need energy, and we need it fast.

Energy

'The only way we can
change our lives is to

change our energy."

DR JOE DISPENZA
AUTHOR AND SCIENTIFIC RESEARCHER

Most mornings, when I wake, it takes me a few moments to gather myself and then I usually check how I feel. Normally, my body feels loose and relaxed. My mind feels open and calm. I feel ready for the day.

Yet that wasn't always the case. Before I discovered the importance of taking time every day to breathe with focus, I used to wake up in a mess. My body used to feel rusty. I was already tired. My mind was cluttered with things to do and people to meet. Before I took my head off the pillow, I was already tired. It wasn't a nice way to start the day.

Then I started to dedicate 10 minutes every day to breathing. Obviously, we breathe all the time. But what I am talking about here is breathing in a certain way. I am talking about taking a few minutes to breathe with focus and intent. When I started to do this, things started to change.

We have already explored how stress and anxiety can affect how we feel. We looked at how focus can help reduce the impact of pressure on us and how that can improve our immunity. We looked at how all of that can improve our performance. So, we have seen how our breath is connected to all our states of mind and body. Included in that is how energetic we feel.

Sometimes, we can feel alive and bursting with energy. Other times, we can be sluggish and tired.

Our levels of energy are affected by many things. We can look at this complex subject from many angles. Are we talking about the intricate relationship between oxygen and our mitochondria (the energy engines in our cells)? Or are we talking about the divine energy that yogis say runs through us and everything in the universe?

Maybe the best approach is to combine a bit of both. To make it simple, let's look at it like this: do you feel that you have the energy to do all the things you need to? Or do you feel you can't do them: you'd prefer to just lie down and have a rest?

Either way, our level of energy affects the quality of our lives. It affects our performance, our mood and our mental health. It affects our relationships. It affects our breathing.

For some people – and I was like this for years when the children were young – it can define us. You'll hear us say: 'I'm wrecked,' and then we'll tell you the full story of why we're so tired. We start to wear it like a badge of honour. It can also become a stick to beat ourselves with.

I met a caring, and open young woman recently. She was studying for exams and working at the same time. When I first met her, there is no way I would have said that she suffered from crippling anxiety. But below the glossy, confident surface, she did. She told me that this was a typical morning for her: after a restless night's sleep, she would wake up and immediately begin to worry about being tired for the rest of the day. She worried that her energy would be low. This made her more anxious, which pushed her up into fight or flight mode. This put her on edge, and her churning mind began to exhaust her. Her day hadn't even started yet.

I have been there too. When our four children were young, my wife Josie and I had years of disturbed sleep. Sometimes we'd have to get up to feed a child or two. Sometimes we'd have to change a nappy in the middle of the night or comfort a sick child. I remember feeling exhausted when I woke up after a night like that. I also remember thinking: 'I'm never going to be able to make it through all those meetings today.' That stress alone was dwindling my fast-depleting energy.

What would happen, though, if I knew how to solve that problem?

What would happen if I knew that I could take 10 minutes to breathe, and it would transform me?

How would that feel?

Well, I can tell you from experience that it feels like liberation.

I began to realise that I could take 10 minutes to breathe, and I would feel relaxed. My mind would settle down. I would let go of all the pressure. I would find a sense of peace. I was no longer in emergency mode. I was floating happily in my rest and recovery mode. When I was there, my body and mind were clear, and they would begin to adapt. My energy would improve. I was no longer struggling.

You can experience that too.

We're going to take a moment to breathe now.

When we begin to breathe, we'll get into a nice rhythm. Then, we'll use our imagination to feel the breath moving up through the body and we'll feel the breath moving down the body. As we breathe in, we'll imagine energy rising through the body with each inhale. Then, we'll imagine letting go of any stress we are holding as we exhale. Then, we'll lengthen our inhales and our holds and our exhales. This will help you ignite your energy.

Unleash the Energy

Take a moment to settle down into a comfortable and safe place, either sitting or lying down.

Let's take two relaxing breaths to begin. Breathe in slowly, and as you exhale, make a sound like a sigh. And again, breathe in slowly and exhale with a sigh.

Rest for a moment.

On your next inhale, breathe in for two and three. Hold your breath now for two and three. Exhale slowly for two and three.

Now, hold your breath for two and three.

Deeply and slowly breathe in for two and three. When you reach the peak of your inhale, hold your breath now for two and three.

Slowly exhale for a count of two and three. Hold this breath now for two and three.

One more time like this...

Breathe in deeply for two and three. Hold the breath for two and three. Exhale slowly for two and three.

Now, hold your breath for two and three.

Take a deep breath in and let go of the exhale. Allow your breathing to find its way back to its natural rhythm.

Let's begin again, and now we're going to use the most powerful tool we have – our imagination.

On your next inhale, imagine energy rising through the body, breathing in for two and three. Now, hold the breath, feeling the energy build as you hold your breath for two and three.

Exhale slowly for two and three, allowing your shoulders to fall and soften. Now stop and hold your breath for two and three.

Breathe in again and imagine your energy rising through the body for a count of two and three. Hold your breath now and feel the energy building and building.

Now exhale slowly with control. Allow any tension you might be holding in your jaw and face to go as you breathe out for two and three.

Hold your breath now for two and three.

Breathe in deeply, feeling your body tingle with the rising energy as you breathe in for two and three. Hold the breath, and the energy, gently pushing it towards the crown of your head and hold for two and three.

Slowly, and with control, release the breath, breathing out for two and three.

Finally, hold this breath for two and three.

As you breathe in now, imagine the energy as a colour (perhaps red, orange or whatever comes to mind) rising through your belly and chest for a count of two, three and four.

Hold your breath now. Feel that colourful, powerful energy build as you hold for two, three and four.

Slowly and with control, begin to exhale, softening your body and breathing out for two, three and four.

Now hold your breath. As you hold, relax your muscles and hold for two, three and four.

Now, breathing in deeply, feel that sparkling energy rising through every cell in the body for two, three and four. At the peak, hold your breath.

Feel the energy gathering in your body as you hold. Continue to hold now for two, three and four.

With control, breathe out slowly for two, three and four.

For the last time, hold your breath. Focus on the sensations within the body, holding your breath for two, three and four.

If you want to, go back to the start of the exercise and begin again. Otherwise, breathe in gently and sigh as you exhale.

Rest now. Allow your breath to find its way back to its natural rhythm. Allow yourself to sink a little deeper into the floor.

Rest for a moment before you go about your day.

Sometimes we believe that we need to rev ourselves up to feel energetic again. But with this exercise, we are changing how we are thinking, going from 'I feel tired' to 'I feel relaxed and rested.' We're allowing ourselves to feel the breath and energy build in us as we hold our breath.

We're releasing tension and stress as we exhale. We're becoming relaxed and alert, energised and focused.

Do this exercise whenever you feel your energy is low. Do it when you want to change how you feel. Do it before you have to do something important that will demand your focus. Do it when you don't feel yourself. As a famous shoemaker often says: just do it.

This way of breathing will calm us down. It will help our minds to settle. Our focus will become more open. We'll start to feel like ourselves again. We'll have the energy we need to do what we have to do.

Sleep

'A good laugh and
a long sleep

are the best cures
for anything."

ANCIENT IRISH PROVERB

There is nothing like a great night's sleep. I love that feeling of waking up refreshed, alert and happy. It is like I've been drifting all night on a calm, dark sea. Usually, I don't remember much: just darkness and the great void. No tossing and turning, no waking up and no having to go to the toilet – just deep sleep.

When I was younger, I always slept well, especially during my basketball days because, of all the training.

But, as our four children started to arrive, one after the other in quick succession, things started to change. For three or four years, Josie and I had to deal with night feeds, nappy changes, teething and midnight escapades nearly every night. As part of that, as a parent, I found that I developed an extrasensory radar system in my mind: I could be asleep, but it felt like I was always listening out for the children: were they okay? Were they waking up? It didn't really turn off. Maybe it was a form of hypervigilance.

Eventually, though, the days, weeks and months passed, and the nights were ours again for sleeping. But I think that radar took a while to shut down – years, maybe. I also noticed that my sleep didn't return to the depth of my nights before children.

But, thankfully, there was a way back to that dark oblivion of a great night's sleep.

I call it the wind-down.

It helps me to shed the tension of the day, to let go of all those churning thoughts and to-do lists, and to slip off into the land of blissful slumber.

What I want to do here is describe how I approach the wind-down and explain the principles behind it. Then, you can take it and adapt it to how you live. You'll find your own version of the wind-down.

There is a point in my evening when I have had enough. I put the laptop away and I throw my phone somewhere. I've had enough technology. I've finished working.

Josie and I then get the children to bed, clean the kitchen and get things ready for the next day. The work for the day is done. That is when the wind-down begins. There is always more work to do, more emails to respond to, but I decide that this is enough for the day.

I described earlier in the book how we used to find sanctuary in our caves and hunted for our lives outside our caves (see page 57). I described how important it is to allow ourselves to feel safe in our cave/sanctuary, and these days, that means reducing the amount of stimulation we are subjected to when we are in our cave.

Well, at this point in the evening, I want to be in my cave. I actually see this as a very important part of our health: winding down from the day and preparing for sleep. I reduce, as much as possible, all the stimulation from technology (screens, phones, social media, etc.). I don't stuff my head full of information from podcasts (although I used to do this all the time). This early stage of the wind-down is to allow my mind time to absorb, and process, the experiences of the day. It is a chance to begin to unwind and slow down.

So, the guiding principle at this point is to reduce all your external stimulation, including technology and stuffing your brain full of more information. It's a time for settling down, quietness and contemplation. This doesn't have to take too long, but it marks a change in the pace of the day.

Although we're focusing here on sleep, you can also use this at other points in the day. Any time you feel overwhelmed, you can take a few minutes to reduce all your incoming stimulation and just sit quietly for a bit.

I often do this when I'm finished cleaning the kitchen for the night. It is a quiet time. I can feel myself shifting down into a lower gear, moving into the parasympathetic nervous system, restoring and healing as this happens.

Then, it is time for the next phase of the wind-down: listening to our breath.

I usually find a comfortable spot on the couch, put a pillow behind my back to keep my spine straight and settle down. I turn off the lights and take a few minutes to enjoy the simple pleasure of sitting down in the dusky evening with nothing to do. After a few moments of this, it is time for The Wrestling Match to begin!

In this comfortable position, I bring my attention to my breath.

Let's do it now.

The Wrestling Match

Slowly place your attention on your breath. Just listen to it. Watch it. Feel it, as it moves through your body. Can you notice your body expanding slightly as you breathe in?

How does your breath feel? Does it feel soft? Or ragged?

Does it feel smooth? Shallow? Deep? Simply observe it as it is now.

Have you noticed something? Have you noticed that by paying attention to it, your breathing starts to change? Sometimes, when we start to pay attention to our breath, we can feel that if we don't continue to pay attention to it, then it might stop! Of course, it won't, but by paying attention to it, we begin to take control of it.

Take a moment or two to continue to watch and listen to your breath.

Now, for the wrestling match!

As you breathe, allow your mind to follow your breath. As you inhale, follow the breath with your attention, and as you exhale, follow it with your attention.

This is your job now: follow your breath with focus and attention. Don't worry about

how you are breathing.
just follow your breath with
your focus.

Sounds easy – and it is, at
the start. But after a few
moments, you'll notice your
thoughts have spun off
somewhere else completely!

So, now, as you read this,
bring your mind back to
your breath. That's it: just
follow your breath as you
inhale. You'll feel your lungs
expanding as you inhale:
simply follow your breath
out as you exhale.

Watch your breath as you
inhale and follow it gently
as you exhale. The reason I
call this a wrestling match is
that without noticing it, your
attention will slip away from
your breath and go running
off into the distance with
some other thought!

So, we have to wrestle our
attention back and put it on
the breath again.

As I sit on my couch doing this, I notice how wild my mind is after an active day. I notice how many thoughts are whizzing around in there. But I just breathe and bring my attention back to each breath. I don't judge myself: 'Hey! You're doing really badly here because you keep losing your focus!' I just wrestle my attention back to my breath. I breathe, pay attention, forget to pay attention, wrestle my mind back to the breath, and continue.

It helps my mind sort through lots of thoughts, emotions and other fluctuations. It is a wrestling match on occasion, but it gives me time to sort through things before I lie down and sleep.

So, this is the guiding principle: taking time to focus on one thing (our breath) allows all the other thoughts and distractions to fall away (even just for a few moments). It helps us process many thoughts and emotions – like cleaning up a disorderly room. Then, we can feel our minds slowing down a little and opening up, and we might find a little more space between our thoughts.

The important thing here is not to be too hard on yourself. This Wrestling Match exercise is about paying attention to your breath and allowing that process to relax us.

Yes, it is difficult at times. But just keep bringing your attention back to your breath. Don't beat yourself up when your mind wanders. There is no right or wrong. No good or bad. There is only breathing and trying to pay attention to it. Take it nice and easy, because this stage of the wind-down is about letting go and unravelling the knotted mind.

I find that I get quite sleepy after this wrestling match. So, I move to the bedroom and lie in bed for the final stage of the wind-down.

The emphasis at this stage is different: I let go of the focus on my breath. The Wrestling Match is over. Instead, I simply focus on breathing softly and calmly. I breathe in for a slow count of four and out for a slow count of four.

Let's do it now.

Surrender to Sleep

Imagine you are lying in your comfortable bed.

Without much effort, breathe in slowly and steadily for a count of two, three and four. Now breathe out gently and slowly for a count of two, three and four.

Feel your belly expand as you breathe in now for a slow count of two, three and four. Breathe out, allowing your body to soften, as you exhale for a count of two, three and four.

Find your rhythm: breathing in slowly for two, three and four. Letting go and breathing out for two, three and four.

Continue to breathe like this for two, three and four. Allowing the body to soften as you breathe out for two, three and four.

As I breathe like this, I feel my mind jump around all over the place at the beginning. But, as I continue, I feel my body soften as I breathe. I feel myself getting heavy, sinking down into the bed as I breathe.

Continue to breathe like this as you begin to drift off into a dream state.

When I first started using the wind-down, part of me was thinking: 'What, another load of things to do before you finally get to bed? Does it ever end?!' But then I realised that I was already doing some version of winding down (for example: listening to a podcast, half-heartedly checking work emails and eventually lying down for a fitful sleep). It was less effective, less soothing and less enjoyable than the wind-down. Most of us have some things we usually do before bed. But replacing those with the wind-down can greatly improve the quality of our sleep.

So, I started to view the wind-down for what it is: a soft and gentle paving of the way to a great night's sleep. It is a little routine that happens when the day's work is done.

As we do these exercises, our bodies begin to let go of the tension of the day. As we listen to our breath, we give the mind permission to sort through those nagging thoughts now, rather than later when our head hits the pillow. As we breathe in this way, we start to feel calm and open.

Then, sleep is just a small step away.

Mood

'When I hear music, I
fear no danger.

I am invulnerable.'

HENRY DAVID THOREAU
AUTHOR AND PHILOSOPHER

My eyes were closed but I could see yellow colours dancing through my mind. I felt divine, floating in space.

But I wasn't in outer space. I was lying on the floor of a training hall in Stroe, in the Netherlands.

It didn't matter, though: nothing mattered. I didn't have a care in the world. We had been breathing deeply for only about 20 minutes, with evocative, rhythmic music playing loudly in the background. Breathing and music make a powerful combination, and this can take us deep into our inner universe. I had gone down into the depths and something startling happened down there.

When I was younger, I was blessed to have four grandparents for the first part of my life. They all lived in Drimnagh, Dublin, an old suburb close to the city. Many people had moved there from the inner city. I had many great memories of them.

Except for my Granny, Vera. In my memories, she was often cold, distant and mean. I could never understand why she behaved like this towards me and my sister and also my parents. I was always deeply conflicted about this: shouldn't your Granny be a lovely old lady? I often used to say: 'I hate her.'

But there on the floor in Stroe, following my breath down

into my inner universe, I realised something profound: my Granny had endured a difficult life. Her beloved husband had died from cancer and left her alone. She was frightened and worried, and money was always a problem. I realised down there in the depths that her worry and fear came out in her behaviour. As well as that, I realised that holding on to my hatred of her had affected my relationships with all the important women in my life (my wife, my sister and my mother). This was a shock to me.

As I lay there, I decided that I had to forgive Vera for what had happened. I began to feel sorry for the hardships she had endured. She was only human, after all, and was trying her best. I decided to love her for all she had done for me. Hell, I wouldn't be here writing this if it wasn't for her! I had never said it before: 'I love you, Vera.'

Simple breathing and music had healed this emotional wound.

I opened my eyes and stared at the ceiling. I stood up and felt lighter. I felt as if a load had been lifted from my shoulders. I looked around at everyone else. Some people were still lying down. Others staring into space. I hugged my friend Isaac who was lying beside me and told him what had happened. He looked a bit shocked. I don't think he had expected this outpouring from me! As we all talked, I realised that everyone in the room had had different experiences. Mine had been profound.

My mood was different as well: lighter, happier. I loved my Granny Vera after all those years and life seemed more colourful and richer because of it.

The next morning, in my hotel room, I decided I wanted to go into the depths again to see what else I could find down there. I took the blankets off the bed and put them on the floor. I lay down on them, settled into a comfortable position and started to breathe.

I learnt another valuable lesson on the floor in the hotel: whenever we take time to breathe, the experience is different. Yes, I wanted to go back down into the depths. But it wasn't going to happen again right away.

Every time we breathe it's different because we are different: it's a different time, our bodies feel different, our mood might be different, and we are different, so the experience of breathing is different.

So, lying on the floor of my hotel room, I enjoyed some blissful breathing. It improved my mood: I felt soothed and delighted. It wasn't as mind-blowing as the previous day, but that was okay. We don't need that experience every time.

This is what I learnt that morning in the hotel and the previous day:

- Breathing, especially when combined with music, can have a deeply therapeutic and healing effect.
- Breathing can change our mood for the better, whenever we need this.
- Every time we take time to breathe, it is different.
- I should let go of my expectations of what I want to happen and just enjoy the experience instead.

So, let's experience that now.

The Music

As you read this, soften your jaw and mouth. Take a moment now to soften the muscles in your shoulders and neck, letting them relax and release.

Now, place your hands on your belly. Or put one hand on your belly and use the other to hold this book!

Either way, breathe in slowly and feel your belly gently expand, then breathe out with a sigh.

Again, breathe in gently, feeling your belly rise and expand, continue breathing to the peak of your inhale and then simply let it go.

Breathe in slowly and softly, feeling your belly expand and breathing to the peak of your inhale, then let go of the breath.

As you breathe like this, there is no tension in the breath; there is no tension in your body.

Breathe in slowly and all the way up to the peak of your inhale. Now, breathe all the way out and down.

Breathe in slowly and up through the body and then when you reach the peak, breathe all the way out.

Your breaths are slow and deep and soft, breathing all

the way in and breathing all the way out.

Find your own pace and rhythm as you breathe. Take it slowly. Take it easy. Enjoy these long inhales and these long exhales. There is no tension in the body as you breathe, no tension in the breath.

Allow your body to soften as you breathe. Again, breathe in slowly, feeling the breath move up through your body to its peak. Now, breathe out, allowing your mind to follow your breath all the way out.

This is the breathing we will use to help improve our mood: full, slow breaths in and full, slow breaths out.

Now, we're going to add music.

Think about the music you love. Music that moves you. Music that brings you joy. That is what we want. We want music that is calming,

uplifting or soothing.

We are going to combine our breathing with that music. We are going to allow the music to lift us, transform us and breathe with us.

There are a few ways to do this. I always think the simplest way is best. So, this is what I suggest you do:

Pick a couple of songs that you like, or a playlist or album. Ideally, find three or four songs. Most songs are usually about three or four minutes long. Just find some music you enjoy and let's start.

The idea is this: you will play the music and breathe for the duration of the three songs. That will be roughly 10 minutes.

Take a moment to find and play your music now.

Click play and let's begin to breathe... As before, place your hands on your belly.

Breathe in slowly and feel your belly gently expand, then breathe out with a sigh.

Breathe in gently again, feeling your belly rise and expand, continue breathing to the peak of your inhale and then simply let it go.

Breathe in slowly and softly, feeling your belly expand and breathing to the peak of your inhale, then let go of the breath.

As you breathe like this, there is no tension in the breath; there is no tension in the body.

One last time like this: breathing in and up through the body until you reach the peak of your inhale, and now just exhale naturally, like a sigh with no forcing.

Rest now for a moment. When we begin to breathe again in a moment, our emphasis will be a little different. We will continue to breathe in and up through the body to the peak of our inhale. But then we will exhale down to the bottom of our exhalation.

So, our breath in is full and deep and our breath out is all the way out. There is no tension in the body or breath. Simply breathing all the way in and all the way out.

Breathe in slowly and all the way up to the peak of your inhale. Now, breathe out slowly and steadily, all the way out and down.

When you reach the bottom of your exhale, begin to breathe back up through the body until you reach the peak of your inhale – and then let go, relax the body, and follow the breath with your mind as you breathe all the way out.

Now, continue to breathe
like this until the end of the
music. The most important
thing is to try to enjoy
each breath.

LET'S BREATHE
TOGETHER

Follow this link to practise
The Music:
www.breathewithniall.com/blissful

We can use The Music exercise any time we are feeling low or unlike ourselves. Take the time to find your music and allow yourself 10 minutes to breathe. I know sometimes taking 10 minutes like this seems like a luxury, but really it is a necessity. This small investment of time is worth the result: at the end of 10 minutes, you'll feel better. The average person spends hours tapping and swiping on their phones every single day. If this is something you recognise, then maybe decide to take a fraction of that time and invest it in improving your mood. It is always worth it.

However, I also know from experience that sometimes we don't have 10 minutes spare. We might be in the middle of something important and we can't just stop and lie down for 10 minutes. In fact, just before I started writing this, I was in the kitchen with Josie. She had a lot going on and was feeling a little low. Right there in the kitchen, we took a couple of minutes to do this simple breathing exercise. It changed the way she was feeling and improved her mood.

For a short exercise that gets quicker results, revisit The Calming Box exercise (see page 72) and spend a couple of minutes doing that. It is a great quick fix.

I often look back at that moment on the floor in the Netherlands when I forgave my Granny as one of the turning points in my life. It freed me from decades of anger and frustration. It liberated me from a prison of my own making and lightened my mood from then on.

Afterwards, I got a lift back into Amsterdam and made my way to the airport. I can't remember if the weather was sunny when I got the train to the airport. But that is how my mood felt. I was light and calm and beaming.

When we combine breathing with beautiful music, we can shake off ways of thinking that may have enslaved us. We can shake off feelings of insecurity and worry. We can shake off morose feelings.

All we have to do is listen to the music and breathe.

Recovery

"There is only one
corner of the universe
you can be certain of
improving.

and that's your own self.'

ALDOUS HUXLEY
ENGLISH WRITER AND PHILOSOPHER

I closed my laptop and lay back on the floor. I stretched my arms above my head and let out a long sigh. I had just guided 200 people through an online breathing masterclass. I love doing these events on Zoom, but it takes a certain type of energy. Especially this session.

The session was for one of the biggest companies in the world. The way this virtual event was set up was a little strange, though: I couldn't see anyone, and they couldn't send me a message (it all came through the host of the event). I could only see my own face on the screen. I knew the audience was out there somewhere, but I had no contact with them.

It didn't help that there was a mix-up with the start time, so I was sitting there, looking at myself on the screen and not knowing if 200 people were watching me too, waiting for me to start. At the agreed time, I started the session, welcoming everyone, talking through what we were going to do. But then I got a direct message from the host – the live stream hadn't started yet. So, I stopped, stared at myself on the screen again and waited. It was a false start.

Eventually, I got the go-ahead and restarted the session; it felt like I was speaking into the void, just me performing into the great silence. It went well in the end, and the client and their staff really enjoyed it. But I felt drained afterwards.

It reminded me of a report I had seen about US military personnel operating attack drones. Years ago, the military assumed that the people operating these drones from their base in the US would not be affected by the actions they were taking (dropping bombs on people). They thought it would be just like playing a computer game and when they were finished, they could just jump in their car and drive home to have dinner with their family. It would be a clean and clinical experience. But life is messy and the operators suffered from stress, anxiety and trauma in the same way they would if they were in battle. It didn't matter that all the action was taking place on a screen: they were human, after all, and the taking of other human lives is traumatic.

This came into my mind as I stared up at the ceiling in the 'sitting lounge' (as the children call our front room). It didn't matter that I had been staring at the screen doing the breathing masterclass; the level of focus, concentration and energy that I used was similar to being onstage, performing in front of lots of people.

This was during the pandemic, and I had another online event shortly afterwards. I needed to recover, and fast.

In my days as an international athlete, I needed to recover quickly as well. Sometimes, at certain basketball tournaments, you could have a game every day (or even twice a day) over a week. Recovery had to be fast and restorative. But, back then, I was stumbling around trying to find answers: I wish I had known what I do now.

Of course, there are many ways to measure recovery. You might be wearing a piece of technology right now (like a smart watch) that will measure all types of bodily functions and tell you if you're on the right path.

These monitoring devices are important, and some people love measuring progress in that way. But I prefer to keep it simple and think we should build up our ability to listen to our bodies. I feel this sensitivity is an essential skill. It is often referred to as interoception: our ability to feel what is going on inside our bodies. For example, we can tell by feeling if our heart is beating too fast or if we are hungry. Like all skills, the more we practise listening to our bodies, the better at it we become.

So, when we are talking about recovery, I like to ask myself a few simple questions to see where I am at that moment:

- Do I feel tense in the body, or loose?
- Do I feel my breathing is soft or ragged?
- Do I feel alert or fuzzy?
- Is my mind clear or cluttered?
- Do I feel like myself?

By asking ourselves these questions, we get a sense of how we are at that moment. So, after my online masterclass, these were my responses:

- My shoulders and neck felt tight.
- My breathing was shallow.
- I felt fuzzy in my brain.
- My mind felt cluttered.
- I felt about 60 per cent myself.

Now, it's your turn.

Let's try it together: as you read on, please answer these questions:

- Do I feel tense in the body, or loose?
- Do I feel my breathing is soft or ragged?
- Do I feel alert or fuzzy?
- Is my mind clear or cluttered?
- Do I feel like myself?

You will know fairly quickly whether you need to spend a little time recovering.

What you are recovering from will be different to me. You might have been running, working late, driving a long distance, answering endless emails. Whatever it is, you'll know where you are after answering these questions.

To help us recover, we are going to combine two types of breathing. They will help us move into the parasympathetic nervous system, allowing us to rest, repair and recover.

How do you know when you have recovered? Well, you'll feel like yourself once more. Of course, you can also go back and answer the questions again to give yourself a sense of how you are feeling.

But, over time, you'll just know that you feel more like yourself.

For some people, this might seem too vague. They might not have a sense of how they feel when they are themselves. So, in that case, I suggest breathing like this for at least 10 minutes. 'Breathing in what way?' I hear you say. Well, let's do it now.

We are going to combine two ways of breathing. I will guide you through it as you read.

We're going to begin with two relaxing breaths...

EXERCISE

The Wave

As you read this, breathe in gently and exhale with a sigh, letting go of any tension in your jaw.

Breathe in again, slowly and softly, and then breathe out, letting go of any tension you feel in your shoulders.

Take a moment now to settle into a comfortable position. Place your attention on your breath as it is now – no forcing or pushing the breath, just watching and listening to it.

On your next inhale, breathe in gently and deeply and then breathe all the way out slowly and steadily.

When you reach the bottom of your exhale, breathe in again – up through the body, feeling it expand as you inhale. Then, without forcing, breathe all the way out. Your exhale is relaxed and soft.

When you get to the bottom of the exhale, breathe in softly and then exhale with a sigh and continue to breathe all the way out slowly.

Rest for a moment now. Allow your breath to return to its natural rhythm. Allow your body to let go of any tension you might be holding, sinking a little deeper into the surface you are on. Rest for a moment.

When we begin again, our emphasis will be a little different.

Our breath in will be deeper, breathing in and up through the body to the peak of the breath. The body will be loose and soft. There will be no tension in the breath. It will move easily and softly through the body.

* So, let's begin again, breathing in deeply and slowly, feeling the body expand and breathing to the peak of your inhale. And now breathing out slowly and down through the body to the bottom of the exhale.

When you get to the bottom of the exhale, breathe in again slowly and steadily up through the body, feeling your breath rising to its peak. And when you get there, let go and breathe out, following your breath with your mind as you breathe all the way out.

When you reach the bottom of the exhale, breathe in steadily and slowly up through the body until you reach the peak. Then, let go, and breathe out and down through the body.

As you breathe in now, imagine your breath as a warm wave rising through you, and when you reach the peak, let go and breathe out and imagine the wave receding, washing down the body as you exhale

Final time...

Breathe in and up through the body, feeling that warm wave rising inside you and moving to its peak.

Let go and feel the wave receding as you breathe all the way out. This is the end of the first round.

Now, go back to the beginning of this exercise (marked with an *) and do two more rounds.

LET'S BREATHE TOGETHER

Follow this link to practise The Wave:
www.breathewithniall.com/blissful

When we are breathing like this, we want our bodies and breath to be soft and easy. Don't worry too much about breathing all the way out, straining yourself in the process. Instead, breathe out for as long as feels comfortable for you. Likewise, on the inhale, feel the body expand as you breathe in and follow the breath up through the body as you continue to breathe, but stay loose and relaxed. Ensure there's no stress or tension as you breathe.

At the end of these rounds, pause for a moment. Allow your breath to rest. Allow your body to really let go.

Allow your mind to open and expand.

How do you feel? Ask yourself these questions again:

- Do I feel tense in the body, or loose?
- Do I feel my breathing is soft or ragged?
- Do I feel alert or fuzzy?
- Is my mind clear or cluttered?
- Do I feel like myself?

If you are feeling more like yourself, then great. If you are not quite there yet, go back to the beginning of the exercise marked with an asterisk and do another few rounds. Breathe like this until you are back to yourself. Then your recovery is complete, and you are ready to take on the day.

One of the strange things I have discovered about recovery is that we often know we need to take time to recover, but we don't do it! When I finished the online masterclass (see page 124), I knew I had to recover quickly, but I still felt resistance to doing something about it. Maybe it is just an Irish attitude – in fact, I often hear people say 'Ah, I'll be grand', meaning that they will just continue as they are even if they don't feel fine.

But, after that masterclass, I knew I had to do something, so I forced myself to breathe like this for 10 minutes. After a few minutes, I could feel my body relax. After a few more minutes, I felt rested, and at the end of 10 minutes, I was back to feeling like myself.

So, use The Wave exercise when you need it.

Making the Blissful Breath Part of You

Breathe until you feel different. Breathe until you are in love with everything!

Breathing makes us feel great. It makes us more patient. It makes us more loving and open. It helps us succeed. It helps us to be ourselves. So, why do we find it so difficult to sit down every day for a few minutes to breathe?

In my work, I share with people my experiences of breathing, the cold, the natural world and the mind. I regularly say: 'A little bit of breathing and a little bit of cold every day – even just a dash of cold at the end of your hot shower – is enough to transform us.' People are often terrified of the cold.

For example, as I was writing this, sitting on the bench in my front garden, a builder walked by and stopped to chat. He knows me, and what I do, and told me he'd never get into the cold – it would kill him! We laughed and he walked on.

Many people feel like this.

But, over many years, I have learnt that the cold isn't the thing people struggle to practise. In the end, they find it easy to fit it into their routine. It's actually the breathing that people struggle with.

I have seen it over and over again. Just last week, I was invited to a beautiful old country estate in Northern Ireland. There, 12 CEOs of successful companies were being guided through the Simple Scaling ScaleX™ Accelerator Programme, which would help them improve and scale their companies. I was there to help them use breathing and the cold to improve their health and clarity of mind as they progressed along the path. After we had spent 30 minutes breathing deeply, I had a conversation with two of the CEOs. It went like this:

CEO 1: 'That was amazing! I feel so relaxed now and clear-headed.'
Me: 'Yeah, taking a few minutes every day to do that is essential.'
CEO 1: 'I find it hard to commit the time to it though.'
CEO 2: 'Think of how much time we spend scrolling on our phones? Reduce that by 10 minutes and there is your time for breathing!'
Me: 'This isn't a luxury, it's a necessity.'

A necessity. An essential part of our day. Not a luxury. Why? Well, as we go about our day, we gather layers and layers of tension within us. It's just a natural reaction to the everyday stresses and strains we encounter.

It's as if we go around gathering up these old coats – each old coat is another layer of stress and tension. After a long day, we are smothered in layer upon layer of stifling old coats, or tension. We need to actively do something to free ourselves from that: to unleash our innate good health, energy and mental clarity. That is where 10 minutes of breathing comes in.

Loads of people I talk to understand why it is important. But they still struggle to find time for it in their day.

I don't think it's a problem with discipline. These people are committed to doing other, more difficult things. I don't think it is a question of not knowing how to do it. These ways of breathing are simple and easy to follow. These people have told me that they know what to do and I have seen them doing it.

So, what the hell is the problem?

After many years, it finally dawned on me one day. You and I are breathing right now as you read this. Our focus on our breath comes and goes. Over the course of our day, we'll breathe about 20,000 times. Most of those breaths go unnoticed – we're too busy doing other stuff. So, our beautiful and hyper-intelligent bodies know that our breathing is being taken care of. We don't need to think about it – it happens automatically.

Other essential things, like eating and drinking, demand our attention: we have to go out and hunt for water and food, otherwise we'll die. Food and water don't just magically appear in front of us.

But breathing is magical; it just happens despite us. This is hardwired into us. So, somewhere deep inside, I feel we don't naturally place much importance on sitting down to breathe for 10 minutes. Somewhere deep inside us, we know we'll do it anyway, so why bother?

Often, recognising the problem is half the battle. Once we realise that we'll naturally dismiss the notion of spending time breathing, then we can anticipate this resistance. Then, we don't have to wonder why we're not doing what we should be doing. Knowing this takes the pressure off a little. It allows us to find a way around the problem. It allows us to adapt to it.

The first part of that is figuring out when to breathe...

Everyone is different. Our lives are different. Our expectations are different. Our schedules are different. So, the time when we breathe with focus should be different, right? Well, sort of. I have coached thousands of people through this process, and this is what I have found:

- Breathing in the morning sets us up for the day. We feel calm, open and ready for whatever happens next.

- Nearly everyone has some type of morning routine (some more rigid than others).

- Setting the alarm 10 minutes earlier than usual can miraculously carve out time for us. And once our 10 minutes of breathing is done, it's done.

- The rest of the day (for me) often gathers momentum and runs away from me. So, I find it easiest to breathe in the morning.

In saying that, though, the mornings may not suit you. The most important thing is to find the spot in the day that works for you. Here are some other times that suit people:

- On a lunch break

- Before a meeting by getting there a few minutes early and breathing in the car or a park beforehand

- After the day's work is done, as part of winding down before bed

Whatever time of day suits you, try to stick with it. Find a little nook of time in the day and repeatedly practise your breathing then. It helps us get into a rhythm, a good habit.

Please avoid this trap, though:

If you are going to set the alarm a bit earlier than usual, get out of bed and do your breathing somewhere else. It is very easy to hit the snooze button and fall back into a deep slumber! I did it many times in the early days and it is incredibly frustrating when you're trying to get into the routine of breathing.

These days, Josie and I set the alarm for 6 a.m. We get up, drink a cup of warm cacao, as part of a little ceremony, then we breathe together. It is a soothing and contemplative start to the day and something I always look forward to. After that, I feel I can handle anything.

Your time spent breathing doesn't have to be a big deal. It doesn't have to take up lots of time. Start with 10 minutes. That's it. If you want to do more, do some more. If you want to do less, grand, do less. The important thing is that you try to do a little every day.

After a while, you will start to crave it.

After a while, time set aside for your breathing practice will become an essential part of your day. After a while, it will be a necessity, not a luxury.

A long time ago, in my previous life working for the charity Concern Worldwide, I had a conversation with an expert from the online betting company Paddy Power. I was trying to figure out how to improve the donation process on the Concern website. At the time, it wasn't an easy donation process – it was asking people too many questions and wasn't easy to follow. The expert from Paddy Power said: 'Don't let them think.' What he meant was that if we have to think about something (such as where do I put my credit card details when donating), then many of us will get confused and that will put us off finishing what we were doing. 'If we confuse them, we lose them' was another catchphrase.

We can apply this to our breathing. This is what I mean. I used to get up early, stumble around looking for clothes to wear, try to sneak downstairs without waking the children up and then try to figure out where I would go to breathe. In the kitchen? No, too dark. In the front room? Too likely to wake the children. Lots of decisions to be made meant that I was confused (especially early in the morning) and more likely to say: 'Oh, forget it,' and go back to bed.

Now, I have taken the thinking, decision-making and confusion out of the experience. I simply get up, pick my clothes up from the floor beside my bed and head straight to the couch downstairs. There are no decisions to make. There is no confusion. I don't have to think, and before I know it, I am downstairs ready to breathe.

Often, practices like this can seem solitary. But really, they work very well when done with other people. During my events, I often have crowds of people sitting or lying down together on beaches, in forests or in sports halls, all breathing together. There is a momentum that builds when we breathe together. There is an energy that gathers. It is a powerful and profound experience.

I once heard Dr Patricia Gerbarg, a psychiatrist and breathwork practitioner, talk about how breathing together, with long, slow exhales when breathing out, activates the vagus nerve, and this stimulates the release of oxytocin, a chemical in the body that helps us bond with each other. I have felt this over and over again – the bond that is created in a room or space when people pause and take time to breathe together.

So, if there is someone special in your life, take some time to sit down with them to breathe. They might not be into it, but you could explain that it would be nice to do it together and help you both find some new (and sacred) common ground. To make it easier, use one of the guided breathing meditations I have recorded for you (you'll find links for these throughout the book). Simply play the audio track, sit back together and follow along. I would recommend doing The Wave breathing (see page 130) on recovery from these guided breathing exercises.

But you don't have to be physically sitting with someone to benefit from this experience. The Covid-19 pandemic has shown us that we can enjoy meaningful relationships remotely through a video conferencing service such as Zoom. I know, I know, many of us are sick of using video services like this. But it is a great way to stay connected. It is also a great way to:

commit to taking 10 minutes every day to breathe

Do it with someone, or with a group online. That accountability can really help to make it a lasting and beneficial habit.

10 Days
of Breathing

Just yesterday, I got a message on Instagram saying that a group of people from all over the world were coming together to do my 10 Days of Breathing Challenge. The challenge is this: to do 10 minutes of breathing every day for 10 days. The great part is that I guide you through the 10 minutes every day. I have recorded 10 different breathing sessions for you. All you need to do is click on the day and follow along. It is the easiest and most effective way to start breathing every day. This group was using WhatsApp to share their experiences and to encourage each other to complete each day of the challenge. When I heard that, I was delighted.

Start the 10 Days of Breathing Challenge now. Just go to: www.breathewithniall.com/blissful.

I am a great believer in people and the wisdom they have within them.

I believe in you. So, experiment with what I have recommended. See what works for you. See what doesn't. You'll find a way that suits you.

I believe that you'll find time to breathe. I believe you'll find a place for it in your day. I believe you'll make blissful breathing a part of you.

The End and Beginning of Your Blissful Breath Journey

The story of the blissful breath started decades ago for me.

Now, I am sitting here in my front room, having just done some deep and blissful breathing. I feel relaxed and open. On the couch across from me are my identical twin girls, reading through a toy catalogue (their favourite 'book') in their soft grey dressing gowns. Upstairs, the rest of the family sleeps soundly.

Never in my wildest dreams did I ever think I would end up here, doing this. Never did I think that I would be able to breathe deeply and clearly without my breath catching in my lungs. Never did I think that my worst weakness (suffering from asthma) would become the focus of my life's work.

Would it be fair to say that the more I mastered my breath, the better my life became?

Would it be fair to say that the more I used my breathing as a force for good, the more open and loving I became?

Would it be fair to say that the more I understood the link between my mind, my breath and my heart, the more successful I became?

Yes, I think all of that is fair.

Across the decades of my life, I have slowly become more aware of my breathing. Eventually, I realised that it was my constant companion. Once I realised that, I started to notice the different qualities of my breathing during different situations.

The more aware I became of my breathing, the more I realised something profound: how I felt was reflected in my breathing. When I realised that I had a choice in how I was breathing, and – because of that – how I was feeling, everything changed.

Imagine for a moment that every time you felt resistance, uncertainty and worry in your day, you were able to change that. You would be able to take a gentle breath in, and breathe out slowly and steadily, and by doing that a few times, the worry would fade away.

Imagine for a moment that every time you were uncertain or fearful, you were able to change that. You were able to bring your attention to your breath in that moment and slow it down, and calmly and evenly breathe in and out, feeling the fear subside.

Imagine for a moment that every time you felt tight and anxious, you were able to change that too. You were able to relax your mouth and jaw. You were able to focus on your breathing and change its rhythm and pace, and by doing so feel safe, calm and open again.

That is what the blissful breath gives us.

How do we get there?

By taking a few minutes every day to sit down and breathe. Put away the emails, the to-do lists and all the rest of it. Just sit down and breathe.

When you feel resistance to doing it, remind yourself that this is a skill. To get good at any skill, we need to practise. But it doesn't have to be a big deal. Just a few minutes. If we're honest with ourselves, we can all find a few minutes each day to invest in something that will dramatically improve our health, our mood and our relationships.

This isn't just any skill, though.

Every part of our lives will improve as we get better at it. Breathing is the beginning and the end of being alive.

At the beginning, we take our first breath and we burst into life.

At the end, we take our last breath and slip into the great unknown.

In between those two breaths (at the beginning and the end), we are constantly inhaling and exhaling. Those breaths are our constant companion. We can ignore them and face the consequences. Or we can work together with them and reap the benefits.

This book can guide you along that path. Use it as a way of finding what works for you.

Use the breathing exercises in this book when you're feeling stressed, when you need to sleep and when you want to recover quickly. This is the end of the book, but it is just the beginning of your mastery.

As you read this now, take a slow, deep breath in and when you reach the peak of your inhale, let go and allow yourself to sigh as you breathe out.

One last time, breathe in gently, inhaling up through your body, and when you reach the peak, just sigh as you breathe out.

That simple movement can change everything.

We can simply, quickly and effectively deal with stress, anxiety and fear.

We can find peace and clarity despite relentless pressure.

We can find deep and profound experiences in the mundane.

The blissful breath is calming and comforting.

The blissful breath is vital and strong.

The blissful breath is restorative and redemptive.

The blissful breath is a force for good in our lives. It helps us. It heals us.

The blissful breath is when we breathe in a way
that transforms us.

Breathe until you feel different.

Breathe until you are in love with everything.

Breathe the blissful breath.

Acknowledgements

First and foremost, thanks to my family for all their support and love. It has never wavered and I appreciate it deeply. As well as my family, I have been blessed, and lucky, to have wise and insightful teachers along the way. Thanks to Grandmaster Shi Yanzi for showing me the importance of discipline and dedication. Thanks to Cáit Branigan for showing me how profound the healing traditions of Ireland are. Thanks to Gina McGarry for showing me that what we need grows around us. Thanks to Wim Hof for showing me how open and loving we can be. Thanks to Dr Richard Brown and Dr Patricia Gerbarg for showing me the healing power of the breath. And finally, a special thanks to Kate Burkett, my editor at Hardie Grant Books, for the encouragement and guidance throughout the writing of this book.

Safety

Always do your breathing exercises in a safe place. If you have any concerns about your health, please consult your doctor before practising.

About the Author

Níall Ó Murchú is a wellness expert with over 20 years' experience. A former international athlete, today Níall teaches people around the world how to use breathing, the cold and nature as forces for good in their lives. Níall's online course 'Blissful Breathing' has helped many people feel calmer and happier despite the stress and pressures they face. If you enjoyed this book, the online course will take your practise deeper. Find out more at www. breathewithniall.com. Níall is based in Dublin, Ireland.

Index

Published in 2022 by Hardie Grant Books,
an imprint of Hardie Grant Publishing

Hardie Grant Books (London)
5th & 6th Floors
52–54 Southwark Street
London SE1 1UN

Hardie Grant Books (Melbourne)
Building 1, 658 Church Street
Richmond, Victoria 3121

hardiegrantbooks.com

All rights reserved. No part of this publication may be
reproduced, stored in a retrieval system or transmitted in any
form by any means, electronic, mechanical, photocopying,
recording or otherwise, without the prior written permission of
the publishers and copyright holders.

The moral rights of the author have been asserted.

Copyright text © Niall Ó Murchú

British Library Cataloguing-in-Publication Data. A catalogue
record for this book is available from the British Library.

The Blissful Breath
ISBN: 9781784885304

10 9 8 7 6 5 4 3 2 1

Publisher: Kajal Mistry
Commissioning Editor: Kate Burkett
Design and Art Direction: Hannah Valentine
Copy-editor: Caroline West
Proofreader: Meredith Olson
Indexer: Cathy Heath
Production Controller: Sabeena Atchia

Colour reproduction by p2d
Printed and bound in China by Leo Paper Products Ltd.

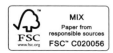